Losing Weight After 50: A Guide to Weight Loss and Maintaining a Healthy Lifestyle

Olive Antoine

DEDICATION

Thanks to my family, especially my niece Glenda, a selfless and diligent soul. To my nephew Nathaniel, my hero, I am blessed to have you in my life. I am thankful for my sister Lady Pearl, and brothers Ricardo and Stanley. My friends Mia, Renya, Philly, Paul, Sean, Rudy, Rachel, Laurel, and Monica, you will always be the "real" ones.
Thank you for your unwavering love and support.

CONTENTS

Contents

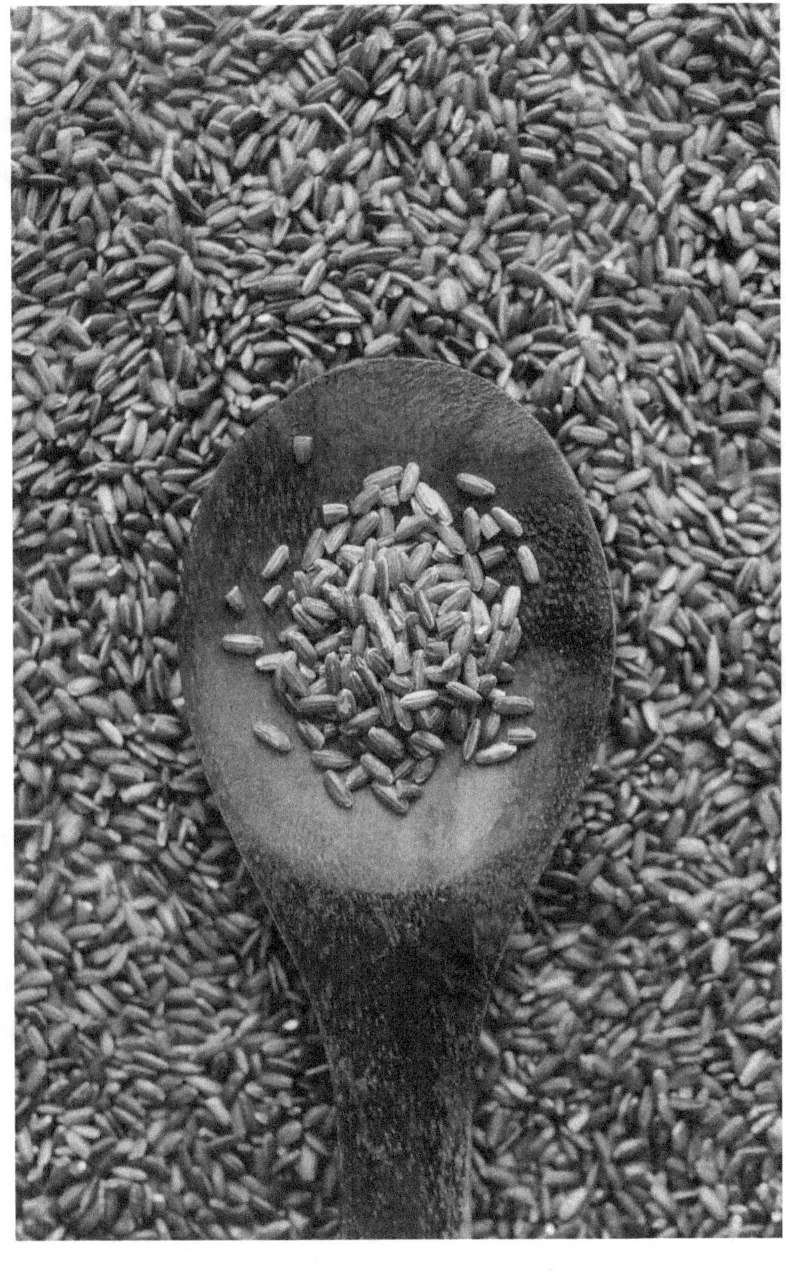

Summary:

In the book "Losing Weight After 50: A Comprehensive Guide to Weight Loss and Maintaining a Healthy Lifestyle," readers are taken on a journey towards achieving weight loss goals and sustaining a healthy lifestyle after the age of fifty. The book covers various aspects that are crucial for success, including understanding the challenges, setting realistic goals, creating a healthy eating plan, engaging in exercise and physical activity, managing stress and sleep, building a support system, overcoming plateaus and challenges, celebrating success, and embracing a healthy lifestyle.

The introduction highlights the unique considerations of losing weight after 50, emphasizing the importance of making sustainable changes and maintaining overall health rather than focusing solely on weight loss. Understanding the challenges provides insights into the physiological and lifestyle factors that may impact weight loss efforts at this stage in life. Setting realistic goals helps readers establish achievable objectives that align with their individual needs and circumstances.

Creating a healthy eating plan guides readers in developing a balanced and sustainable approach to nutrition, emphasizing whole, nutrient-dense foods while allowing for occasional indulgences. The chapter on exercise and physical activity encourages readers to engage in a variety of activities that they enjoy, promoting cardiovascular health, strength, and flexibility. Managing stress and sleep highlights the significance of these factors in weight loss and provides practical strategies for effective stress management and quality sleep.

Building a support system emphasizes the importance of seeking support from loved ones, joining weight loss groups or online communities, and consulting professionals who specialize in weight loss for individuals over fifty. Overcoming plateaus and challenges offers strategies for breaking through weight loss plateaus and staying motivated during tough times.

Celebrating success and maintaining weight loss focuses on acknowledging and rewarding achievements while implementing strategies to sustain progress. Embracing a healthy lifestyle encompasses adopting a comprehensive approach to health, encompassing nutrition, physical activity, stress management, relationships, and mindset. It encourages readers to prioritize self-care, practice gratitude, and cultivate positive habits for long-term well-being.

Overall, "Losing Weight After 50: A Comprehensive Guide to Weight Loss and Maintaining a Healthy Lifestyle" provides readers with practical advice, strategies, and insights to support their weight loss journey and help them lead a healthy and fulfilling life beyond their weight loss goals.

Introduction

Chapter 1: Introduction to Losing Weight After 50

Once we cross the age of fifty, our bodies undergo various changes that can make losing weight a bit challenging. However, with the right knowledge, determination, and a comprehensive plan, losing weight and maintaining a healthy lifestyle is entirely achievable. In this book, we will explore the essential strategies, tips, and techniques specifically designed for individuals over fifty who are looking to shed those extra pounds and embark on a healthier journey.

Chapter 2: Understanding the Challenges

Before diving into the weight loss journey, it is crucial to understand the challenges that come with losing weight after 50. Hormonal changes, decreased metabolism, muscle loss, and a sedentary lifestyle are some of the factors that can affect weight management. By acknowledging and addressing these challenges, you will be better equipped to make effective and sustainable changes.

Chapter 3: Setting Realistic Goals

Setting realistic and achievable goals is a vital step in any weight loss journey. In this chapter, we will discuss the importance of setting specific, measurable, attainable, relevant, and time-bound (SMART) goals. We will guide you through the process of establishing realistic targets that align with your body's capabilities and help you stay motivated throughout the journey.

Chapter 4: Creating a Healthy Eating Plan

Diet plays a significant role in weight loss, regardless of age. However, after 50, it becomes even more crucial to adopt a balanced and nutritious eating plan. In this chapter, we will explore different dietary approaches, such as portion control, mindful eating, and focusing on whole foods. We will also discuss the importance of hydration and the role of supplements in supporting weight loss.

Chapter 5: Exercise and Physical Activity

Regular physical activity is essential for weight loss and overall health. But after 50, it is important to choose exercises that suit your body and lifestyle. In this chapter, we will discuss low-impact exercises, strength training, and flexibility exercises that are suitable for individuals over fifty.

We will also explore the benefits of incorporating physical activity into your daily routine and provide.

Tips for staying motivated.

Chapter 6: Managing Stress and Sleep

Stress and lack of sleep can sabotage your weight loss efforts. In this chapter, we will delve into stress management techniques, including meditation, deep breathing exercises, and finding healthy outlets for stress. We will also discuss the importance of quality sleep and provide practical tips for improving your sleep hygiene.

Chapter 7: Building a Support System

Having a support system can make a world of difference in your weight loss journey. In this chapter, we will discuss the importance of building a support network of family, and friends, or joining communities or groups that share similar goals. We will also explore the benefits of accountability partners and how they can help you stay on track.

Chapter 8: Overcoming Plateaus and Challenges

Weight loss plateaus and challenges are common, but they should not deter you from reaching your goals. In this chapter, we will discuss strategies to overcome plateaus, including modifying your exercise routine, adjusting your calorie intake, and exploring new activities.

We will also address shared challenges faced by individuals over fifty and provide solutions to help you stay focused.

Chapter 9: Celebrating Success and Maintaining Weight Loss

Reaching your weight loss goals is a remarkable achievement. However, the journey does not end there. In this chapter, we will explore strategies for maintaining weight loss, including mindful eating, regular exercise, and developing healthy habits for the long term. We will also discuss the importance of celebrating your success and rewarding yourself along the way.

Chapter 10: Embracing a Healthy Lifestyle

Losing weight after 50 is not just about shedding pounds; it is about embracing a healthy lifestyle. In this closing chapter, we will explore how to make lasting changes that go beyond weight loss and focus on overall well-being.

We will delve into the importance of finding joy in physical activity and discovering activities that you truly enjoy. Additionally, we will discuss nurturing healthy relationships and the impact they can have on your mental and emotional well-being.

Self-care and self-compassion will also be emphasized, as taking care of yourself is essential for long-term success. By the end of this chapter, you will have the tools and knowledge to create a balanced and fulfilling lifestyle that supports your weight loss journey and promotes a healthier, happier you.

Chapter 1: Introduction to Losing Weight After 50

Once we cross the age of 50, our bodies undergo various changes that can make losing weight a bit challenging. It's important to approach weight loss after 50 with a different perspective and understanding of how our bodies function at this stage of life. Hormonal shifts, decreased metabolism, muscle loss, and a sedentary lifestyle are some of the factors that can affect weight management.

Hormonal changes, such as menopause in women, can cause shifts in body composition and lead to weight gain, particularly around the midsection. This is because the decrease in estrogen levels affects the way our bodies store fat.

Additionally, men also experience a decline in testosterone levels, which can contribute to reduced muscle mass and slower metabolism.

Another challenge that individuals over 50 face is a decrease in metabolic rate. As we age, our bodies naturally burn fewer calories at rest, making it more difficult to create a calorie deficit for weight loss.

This means that the strategies we may have used in our younger years, such as simply reducing portion sizes or increasing physical activity, may not yield the same results.

Furthermore, muscle loss, known as sarcopenia, becomes more prevalent after the age of 50. This loss of muscle mass not only affects strength and mobility but also contributes to a decrease in metabolic rate. Since muscle tissue burns more calories than fat, a reduction in muscle mass can further slow down weight loss progress.

Additionally, the sedentary lifestyle that many individuals lead after 50 can hinder weight loss efforts. With retirement and fewer work-related physical activities, it's important to make a conscious effort to incorporate regular exercise into daily routines.

Finding enjoyable activities that promote movement and strength training becomes crucial in maintaining a healthy weight.

Despite these challenges, it's important to remember that losing weight after 50 is entirely possible with the right approach. By understanding the changes our bodies go through and tailoring our strategies accordingly, we can achieve our weight loss goals and embark on a healthier journey.

Throughout this book, we will explore effective strategies, tips, and techniques designed specifically for individuals over 50, empowering you to take control of your health and well-being.

Chapter 2: Understanding the Challenges

Before diving into the weight loss journey, it's crucial to understand the challenges that come with losing weight after 50. By recognizing and addressing these challenges, you can develop a realistic and effective plan to overcome them.

One of the primary challenges of losing weight after 50 is hormonal changes. In women, the transition into menopause brings about hormonal fluctuations, particularly a decrease in estrogen levels. This hormonal shift can lead to changes in body composition, including an increase in abdominal fat. It can also affect mood, energy levels, and metabolism.

Understanding how these hormonal changes impact weight gain and metabolism is essential for designing an effective weight loss strategy.

Another challenge is the decrease in metabolic rate. As we age, our bodies naturally burn fewer calories at rest. This reduction in basal metabolic rate makes it more difficult to create a calorie deficit, which is essential for weight loss.

 It means that the approaches that may have worked in the past, such as simply reducing portion sizes, may no longer be sufficient.

Understanding the relationship between age, metabolism, and calorie balance will help you tailor your approach to achieving weight loss success.

Muscle loss, known as sarcopenia, is another significant challenge. As we age, our bodies tend to lose muscle mass, which can lead to a decrease in strength, mobility, and metabolic rate. The loss of muscle mass also makes it more challenging to burn calories and maintain a healthy weight.

To combat muscle loss, incorporating regular strength training exercises becomes crucial. Strength training not only helps preserve muscle mass but also improves bone density, balance, and overall functional fitness.

Moreover, a sedentary lifestyle often becomes more prevalent after 50. With retirement or fewer work-related physical activities, it's easier to slip into a sedentary routine.

However, a lack of physical activity can hinder weight loss efforts and contribute to muscle loss and decreased metabolism. It's important to adopt an active lifestyle by incorporating regular exercise and movement into your daily routine. Finding activities you enjoy, such as walking, swimming, cycling, or group classes, can help you stay motivated and consistent with your exercise routine.

By understanding these challenges, you can develop strategies that specifically address them. It's important to approach weight loss after 50 with patience, persistence, and a comprehensive plan that considers hormonal changes, metabolic slowdown, muscle loss, and a sedentary lifestyle.

In the upcoming chapters, we will explore strategies and techniques tailored to these challenges, empowering you to overcome them and achieve your weight loss goals.

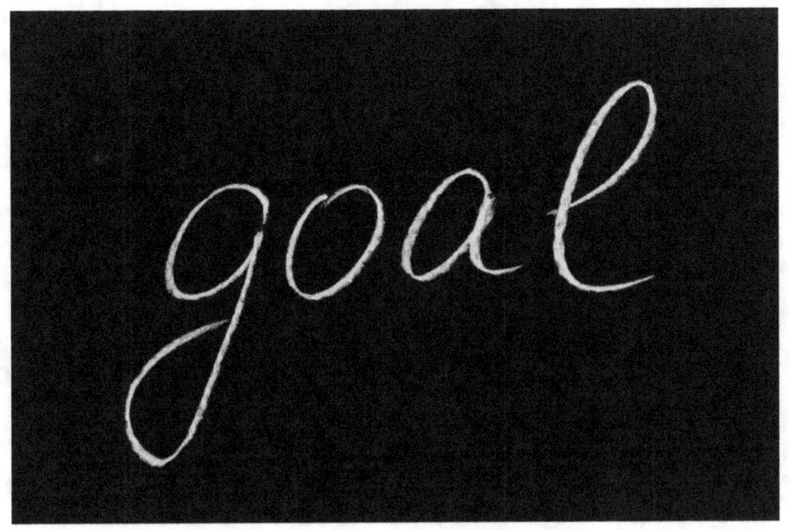

Chapter 3: Setting Realistic Goals

Setting realistic and achievable goals is a vital step in any weight loss journey, particularly when you're over 50. By setting specific, measurable, attainable, relevant, and time-bound (SMART) goals, you can establish a clear path toward success while maintaining a realistic perspective.

Firstly, it's essential to set specific goals that clearly define what you want to achieve. Instead of stating a vague goal like "lose weight," specify the amount of weight you aim to lose.

For example, setting a goal to lose 10 pounds in three months provides a clear target to work towards. Specific goals enable you to track your progress more effectively and stay motivated along the way.

Measurable goals allow you to track your progress and provide a sense of accomplishment as you reach milestones. Instead of focusing solely on the number on the scale, consider incorporating other measurements such as waist circumference, body fat percentage, or clothing sizes. These measurable markers can indicate progress even when the scale may not reflect it accurately.

Setting attainable goals is crucial for maintaining motivation and avoiding disappointment. While it's important to challenge yourself, setting unrealistic goals can lead to frustration and discouragement. Consider factors such as your current health status, lifestyle, and time commitments when determining what is attainable for you. It's better to set smaller, achievable goals that can be consistently met and build momentum over time.

Relevance is another key factor in goal setting. Ensure that your goals align with your overall health and well-being. Consider why losing weight is important to you and how it will positively impact your life.

This personal relevance will help you stay focused and committed to your goals, especially when faced with challenges.

Lastly, incorporating a time-bound aspect to your goals adds a sense of urgency and accountability. Set a realistic timeline for achieving your weight loss goals, considering factors such as your metabolism, lifestyle, and the recommended rate of weight loss. This time frame can serve as a benchmark and keep you on track throughout your journey.

Remember that weight loss is not solely about reaching a specific number on the scale. It's also about improving your overall health, well-being, and quality of life.

Setting realistic goals that are specific, measurable, attainable, relevant, and time-bound will help you maintain focus, celebrate milestones, and sustain motivation throughout your weight loss journey. In the upcoming chapters, we will explore strategies to help you achieve these goals and create lasting changes for a healthier lifestyle.

Chapter 4: Creating a Healthy Eating Plan

Diet plays a significant role in weight loss, regardless of age. However, when you're over 50, it becomes even more crucial to adopt a balanced and nutritious eating plan that suits your body's changing needs. In this chapter, we will explore the key elements of creating a healthy eating plan to support your weight loss goals and overall well-being.

One important aspect of a healthy eating plan is portion control. As we age, our metabolism tends to slow down, meaning we require fewer calories to maintain our weight. It's essential to pay attention to portion sizes and ensure they align with your body's energy needs.

Using measuring cups, portion control plates, or visual cues can help you gauge appropriate portion sizes and avoid overeating.

Mindful eating is another valuable strategy to incorporate into your eating plan. By slowing down, savoring each bite, and paying attention to hunger and fullness cues, you can develop a healthier relationship with food. Mindful eating encourages you to listen to your body's signals and eat when you're hungry, rather than relying on external cues or emotional triggers.

Focusing on whole foods is crucial for a nutritious eating plan. Whole foods, such as fruits, vegetables, whole grains, lean proteins, and healthy fats, are rich in essential nutrients, fiber, and antioxidants. These foods provide nourishment and support your overall health while helping you feel satisfied and energized. Aim to include a variety of colorful fruits and vegetables, lean proteins like poultry, fish, legumes, and whole grains in your meals.

Hydration is often overlooked but plays a vital role in weight loss and overall well-being. Drinking an adequate amount of water helps maintain proper bodily functions, supports digestion, and can even aid in appetite control.

Make it a habit to drink water throughout the day and consider replacing sugary beverages with water or herbal teas to reduce unnecessary calorie intake. In addition to a well-rounded diet, supplements may be beneficial, especially for individuals over 50. As we age, certain nutrients may become more challenging to absorb or obtain from food alone.

Consult with a healthcare professional to determine if supplements such as vitamin D, calcium, or omega-3 fatty acids are suitable for you based on your specific needs.

It's important to remember that a healthy eating plan should not feel restrictive or overly complicated. Strive for balance and moderation, allowing yourself the flexibility to enjoy occasional treats or indulge in social gatherings.

It's not about perfection but rather making sustainable, long-term changes to your eating habits that support your weight loss goals and overall health.

In the upcoming chapters, we will delve deeper into specific dietary approaches, meal planning, and practical tips to help you implement and maintain a healthy eating plan.

By nourishing your body with wholesome foods, practicing portion control, and adopting mindful eating habits, you will be on your way to achieving weight loss success and enjoying a healthier lifestyle.

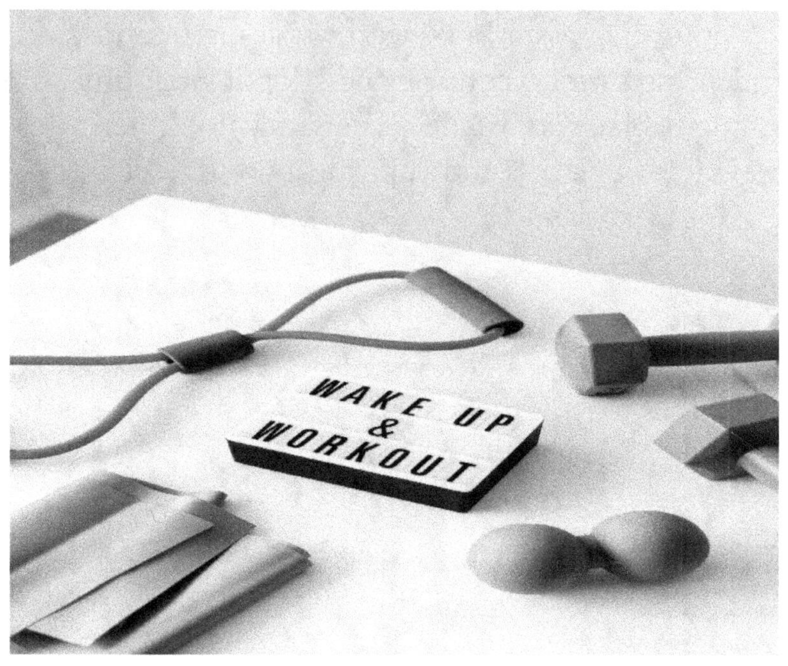

Chapter 5: Exercise and Physical Activity

Regular physical activity is essential for weight loss and overall health, especially as we age. Engaging in exercise and physical activity can help you burn calories, build strength, improve cardiovascular health, and enhance your overall well-being. In this chapter, we will explore exercise strategies specifically tailored for individuals over 50 to support weight loss and maintain a healthy lifestyle.

When it comes to exercise, it's important to choose activities that suit your body and lifestyle. Low-impact exercises, such as walking, swimming, cycling, or using an elliptical machine, can be gentle on your joints while still providing effective cardiovascular benefits. These activities can be easily incorporated into your daily routine and can be enjoyable and sustainable in the long run.

Strength training is particularly important for individuals over 50. As we age, we naturally lose muscle mass, which can lead to a decrease in metabolic rate and a reduction in strength and mobility. By incorporating regular strength training exercises, such as using resistance bands, lifting weights, or practicing bodyweight exercises, you can help preserve and build muscle mass.

Strength training not only boosts your metabolism but also improves bone density, balance, and functional fitness, reducing the risk of falls and maintaining overall strength and mobility.

Flexibility exercises, such as stretching, yoga, or Pilates, are also beneficial for individuals over 50. These activities help improve joint range of motion, enhance flexibility, and promote better posture. They can also aid in relaxation and stress reduction, which is crucial for overall well-being.

Finding activities, you enjoy is key to maintaining consistency and motivation. Consider joining group fitness classes, such as aerobics, dance, or yoga classes, where you can socialize and make exercise a fun and social experience. Alternatively, explore outdoor activities like hiking, gardening, or golfing. The key is to find activities that you look forward to and that fit your lifestyle, so you are more likely to stick with them in the long term.

In addition to structured exercise sessions, it's important to incorporate more movement into your daily routine. This can include simple changes such as taking the stairs instead of the elevator, walking or biking instead of driving for short distances or incorporating short bouts of physical activity during breaks at work. These small changes can add up and contribute to increased calorie expenditure and overall physical fitness.

It's worth noting that before starting any new exercise program, it's advisable to consult with a healthcare professional, particularly if you have any pre-existing medical conditions or concerns. They can provide guidance and ensure you engage in activities that are safe and appropriate for your individual needs.

In the upcoming chapters, we will delve deeper into specific exercise routines, tips for staying motivated, and strategies for incorporating physical activity into your daily life. By choosing activities that suit your body, focusing on strength training, flexibility, and finding enjoyment in exercise, you'll be well on your way to achieving your weight loss goals and maintaining a healthy lifestyle.

Chapter 6: Managing Stress and Sleep

When it comes to weight loss and maintaining a healthy lifestyle, managing stress, and prioritizing quality sleep are often overlooked but essential components. As we age, stress levels can increase, and sleep patterns may become disrupted, making it crucial to develop strategies to effectively manage stress and promote restful sleep. In this chapter, we will explore the importance of stress management and sleep and provide practical tips for incorporating them into your weight loss journey.

Stress management is essential because high levels of stress can contribute to weight gain and hinder weight loss efforts. When we're stressed, our bodies release cortisol, a hormone that can increase appetite, especially for high-calorie and sugary foods. Additionally, stress can lead to emotional eating or a decrease in motivation to engage in physical activity.

Therefore, finding effective ways to manage stress is vital for maintaining a healthy lifestyle. Engaging in stress-reducing activities, such as meditation, deep breathing exercises, or yoga, can help calm the mind and relax the body. These practices can lower cortisol levels, promote a sense of well-being, and improve overall mental and emotional health.

Find a technique that resonates with you and incorporate it into your daily routine, even if it's for just a few minutes. Prioritizing self-care activities, such as taking a bath, reading a book, or engaging in a hobby you enjoy, can also be effective in managing stress levels.

Another crucial aspect of overall well-being and weight management is getting adequate sleep. Sleep plays a vital role in regulating hormones that affect appetite and metabolism.

Insufficient sleep can disrupt these hormonal processes, leading to increased hunger, cravings,

and a decrease in the sensation of fullness.

It can also negatively impact energy levels and motivation to engage in physical activity.

To promote better sleep, establish a regular sleep schedule and create a relaxing bedtime routine. Aim to go to bed and wake up at the same time each day, even on weekends. Create a soothing environment in your bedroom by keeping it cool, dark, and quiet. Limit exposure to electronic devices, especially before bedtime, as the blue light emitted by screens can interfere with sleep quality.

Implementing relaxation techniques, such as gentle stretching, deep breathing, or reading a book, before bed can help signal to your body that it's time to unwind and prepare for sleep. Avoid consuming caffeine, alcohol, and large meals close to bedtime, as they can disrupt sleep patterns. Instead, opt for a light snack if necessary, such as a small portion of protein or a piece of fruit.

Additionally, incorporating regular physical activity into your routine can positively impact both stress management and sleep quality. Exercise can help reduce stress levels, promote relaxation, and improve sleep.

However, it's important to avoid intense workouts too close to bedtime, as they can elevate energy levels and make it difficult to wind down. By managing stress effectively and prioritizing quality sleep, you can support your weight loss efforts and overall well-being. Incorporate stress-reducing activities into your daily routine, establish a

relaxing bedtime routine and create a sleep-friendly.

environment. As you navigate the upcoming chapters, you'll discover more strategies to help you effectively manage stress and improve sleep, enabling you to achieve your weight loss goals and maintain a healthy lifestyle.

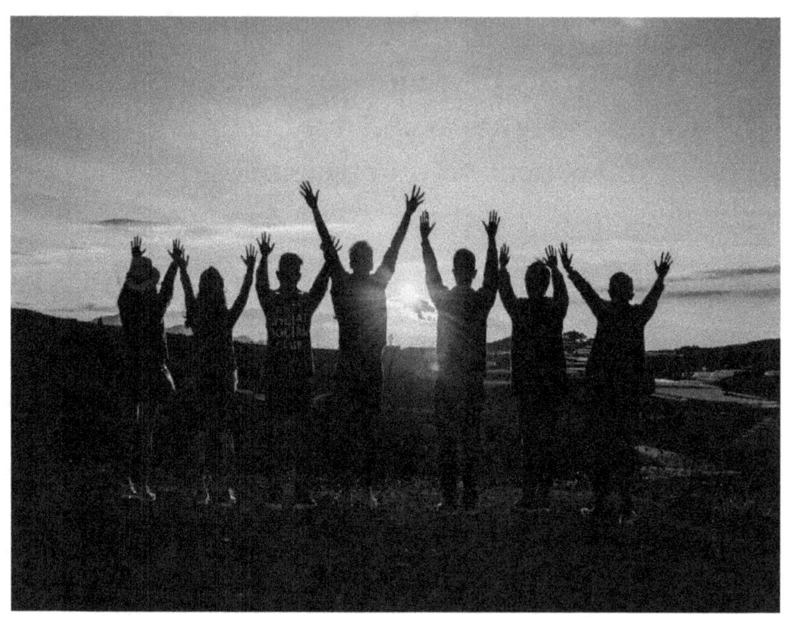

Chapter 7: Building a Support System

Embarking on a weight loss journey after 50 can be challenging, but having a strong support system can make a significant difference in your success. Building a support network of family, friends, and like-minded individuals can provide the encouragement, accountability, and motivation needed to stay on track and overcome obstacles.

In this chapter, we will explore the importance of a support system and provide guidance on how to build one that suits your needs.

Having support from loved ones is invaluable. Share your weight loss goals and intentions with your family and close friends. Explain to them why it's important to you and how their support can make a difference. Communicate your needs and enlist their encouragement, understanding, and assistance. Having a network of individuals who believe in your journey and cheer you on can provide the emotional boost needed during challenging times.

Consider finding a weight loss buddy or joining a support group. Having someone who is on a similar path can provide additional motivation, accountability, and a sense of camaraderie. Look for local weight loss groups or online communities where you can connect with individuals who share similar goals. These groups often offer a platform for sharing experiences, seeking advice, and celebrating milestones together.

Seeking professional support is also beneficial. Consult with a registered dietitian, nutritionist, or weight loss coach who specializes in working with individuals over 50.

They can provide personalized guidance, help you develop a customized eating plan, and offer strategies tailored to your specific needs. Additionally, consider working with a personal trainer or exercise professional who can design a safe and effective exercise program based on your abilities and goals.

Technology can be an excellent tool for building and maintaining a support system. There are numerous weight loss apps, online forums, and virtual communities that can provide guidance, track your progress, and offer support. These platforms allow you to connect with individuals from around the world who are also on their weight loss journey, offering a sense of community and shared experiences.

Remember that building a support system is a two-way street. Be willing to offer support and encouragement to others who may be on their own weight loss journey. By being a source of motivation and inspiration for others, you can strengthen your commitment and reinforce positive behaviors within yourself.

Lastly, if you find that your current support system is not as supportive as you need it to be, consider seeking out additional resources.

Look for local wellness programs, community centers, or support groups specifically designed for individuals over 50. These programs often provide education, resources, and a supportive environment to help you achieve your weight loss goals.

In conclusion, building a support system is vital for successful weight loss after 50.

Surround yourself with individuals who believe in you, connect with like-minded individuals through weight loss groups or online communities, seek professional guidance, and utilize technology to enhance your support network. With the support and encouragement of others, you'll find the strength and motivation to overcome challenges, celebrate achievements, and maintain a healthy lifestyle for years to come.

Chapter 8: Overcoming Plateaus and Challenges

During your weight loss journey, it's common to encounter plateaus and face various challenges that may test your determination. However, with the right strategies and mindset, you can overcome these obstacles and continue making progress toward your goals. In this chapter, we will explore effective ways to overcome plateaus and navigate through common challenges that arise when losing weight after 50.

Plateaus occur when your weight loss progress stalls and it can be frustrating. However, it's important to remember that plateaus are a normal part of the process and shouldn't discourage you. Instead, use them as an opportunity to reassess and adjust your approach.

One strategy to overcome plateaus is to evaluate your eating and exercise habits. Consider whether you have become too comfortable with your routine and if there are any areas where you can make improvements.

Fine-tuning your eating plan by reducing portion sizes, increasing nutrient-dense foods, or adjusting macronutrient ratios can help jump-start your progress. Similarly, modifying your exercise routine by incorporating new activities, increasing intensity, or trying different workout formats can challenge your body and help break through a plateau.

It's essential to stay committed and consistent, even during challenging times. Set realistic expectations and remind yourself that sustainable weight loss takes time.

Avoid comparing your progress to others and focus on your own journey. Celebrate small victories along the way, such as improvements in strength, endurance, or overall well-being, which may not always be reflected in the numbers on the scale.

Another common challenge is maintaining motivation. As you progress on your weight loss journey, it's natural for motivation to fluctuate.

During periods when motivation is low, remind.

yourself of your initial reasons for wanting to lose weight and the benefits you have experienced thus far.

Revisit your goals and adjust them if necessary.

to ensure they continue to align with your values and aspirations.

Seeking support from your network can also be instrumental in overcoming challenges. Lean on your support system, whether it's family, friends, or a weight loss group, for encouragement and accountability.

Share your struggles and successes with them, and they can provide the motivation and perspective you need to keep going.

Mindset plays a crucial role in overcoming challenges. Adopt a positive and growth-oriented mindset, viewing obstacles as opportunities for learning and growth. Rather than seeing setbacks as failures, consider them as valuable feedback to refine your approach and improve your strategies.

Embrace a mindset of self-compassion and kindness, recognizing that setbacks are part of the journey and do not define your worth or potential for success.

Additionally, focusing on non-scale victories can be.

empowering and help you stay motivated. Notice the positive changes in your body, such as improved energy levels, better sleep, increased flexibility, or enhanced mood. Celebrate these achievements and use them as reminders of how far you've come.

In conclusion, overcoming plateaus and challenges is an integral part of your weight loss journey. Embrace plateaus as opportunities to reassess and adjust, stay committed and consistent, seek support from your network, maintain a positive mindset, and focus on non-scale victories.

With resilience, determination, and the right strategies, you can overcome any obstacles that come your way and continue making progress towards your weight loss goals after 50.

Chapter 9: Celebrating Success and Maintaining Weight Loss

Reaching your weight loss goals is a significant achievement, but the journey doesn't end there. Celebrating your success and implementing strategies to maintain your weight loss is essential for long-term success and a healthy lifestyle. In this chapter, we will explore the importance of celebrating milestones and provide practical tips for maintaining your weight loss after reaching your goals.

Celebrating your success is more than just a way to reward yourself—it's a way to acknowledge and appreciate the hard work and dedication you've put into your weight loss journey. Take the time to reflect on how far you've come, both physically and mentally. Celebrate each milestone, whether it's reaching a specific weight, fitting into a smaller clothing size, or achieving a personal fitness goal. Treat yourself to something special, such as a new outfit, a spa day, or a weekend getaway, as a tangible reminder of your accomplishments.

Maintaining your weight loss requires a shift in mindset and lifestyle. Instead of viewing it as a temporary endeavor, adopt the mindset that weight management is an ongoing process. Recognize that the habits and behaviors you developed during your weight loss journey should continue as part of your daily routine.

One crucial strategy for maintaining weight loss is to establish a balanced and sustainable eating plan. Continue to prioritize whole, nutrient-dense foods while allowing yourself occasional indulgences in moderation. Aim for a balanced macronutrient ratio that suits your individual needs and preferences. Focus on portion control and mindful eating, paying attention to hunger and fullness cues.

Regularly evaluate your eating habits and adjust as needed to ensure you're nourishing your body while maintaining a healthy weight.

Physical activity remains an integral component of weight maintenance. Continue to engage in regular exercise and find activities you enjoy. Aim for a combination of cardiovascular exercise, strength training, and flexibility exercises to support overall fitness and well-being.

Consider setting new fitness goals to stay motivated and challenged.

This could involve participating in a local charity run, joining a sports league, or trying out new fitness classes that pique your interest.

Regular monitoring and self-awareness are key to maintaining weight loss. Keep track of your weight, body measurements, and energy levels. Regularly assess your eating and exercise habits to ensure you're staying on track. If you notice any changes, such as gradual weight gain or slipping into old habits, take proactive steps to address them. Seek support from your network, whether it's family, friends, or a support group, to help you stay accountable and motivated.

Mindful eating and managing emotional triggers are crucial for maintaining weight loss.

Be mindful of your eating habits, pay attention to hunger and fullness cues, and avoid mindless snacking or emotional eating. Develop alternative coping mechanisms for stress or emotional triggers, such as engaging in relaxation techniques, practicing self-care activities, or seeking support from loved ones.

Building a healthy relationship with food and addressing emotional eating patterns can greatly contribute to long-term weight maintenance.

Lastly, practice self-compassion and kindness

throughout your weight maintenance journey. Accept that there will be fluctuations and challenges along the way.

Be patient with yourself and celebrate progress, even if it's not always perfect. Surround yourself with positive influences and remind yourself of your worth beyond your weight or appearance.

In conclusion, celebrating your success and implementing strategies for weight maintenance are essential for long-term success and a healthy lifestyle. Take the time to acknowledge and celebrate your achievements, shift your mindset towards ongoing weight management, maintain a balanced eating plan, continue regular physical activity, monitor your progress, practice mindful eating, and be kind to yourself throughout the process. By implementing these strategies, you can enjoy the rewards of your hard work and maintain a healthy weight for years to come.

Chapter 10: Embracing a Healthy Lifestyle

Achieving weight loss goals after 50 goes beyond simply shedding pounds. It's about embracing a healthy lifestyle that promotes overall well-being and vitality. In this chapter, we will delve into the importance of adopting a holistic approach to health and provide practical tips for embracing a healthy lifestyle.

Embracing a healthy lifestyle means making conscious choices that benefit your physical, mental, and emotional well-being. It involves nurturing your body with nutrient-dense foods, engaging in regular physical activity, managing stress effectively, prioritizing self-care, and fostering positive relationships and connections.

Nutrition plays a fundamental role in a healthy lifestyle. Focus on consuming a variety of whole, unprocessed foods, such as fruits, vegetables, lean proteins, whole grains, and healthy fats. Strive for a balanced and colorful plate that provides essential vitamins, minerals, and antioxidants. Avoid highly processed and sugary foods as much as possible, as they can contribute to weight gain and negatively impact overall health. Listen to your body's hunger and fullness cues, and eat mindfully, savoring each bite and being present during meals.

Regular physical activity is vital for maintaining a healthy lifestyle. Aim for a combination of cardiovascular exercise, strength training, and flexibility exercises. Find activities that you enjoy and can incorporate into your routine consistently. Whether it's brisk walking, cycling, swimming, dancing, or participating in group fitness classes, choose activities that keep you engaged and motivated. Remember, the goal is not just weight loss but overall fitness, strength, and endurance.

Stress management is a crucial aspect of a healthy lifestyle. Chronic stress can have detrimental effects on your physical and mental well-being, contributing to weight gain, increased risk of chronic diseases, and reduced quality of life.

Explore stress-reducing techniques such as mindfulness meditation, deep breathing exercises, yoga, or engaging in hobbies and activities that.

bring you joy and relaxation. Prioritize self-care and carve out time for activities that nourish your soul and promote a sense of calm and balance.

Nurturing positive relationships and connections is an essential component of a healthy lifestyle. Surround yourself with supportive and like-minded individuals who uplift and inspire you. Cultivate meaningful connections with family, friends, and community members who share similar values and goals. Engage in social activities, volunteer work, or join clubs and organizations that align with your interests. Building a strong support network and maintaining healthy relationships can greatly enhance your overall well-being and contribute to long-term success.

In addition to nutrition, physical activity, stress management, and relationships, prioritizing sleep is paramount for a healthy lifestyle. Aim for 7-9 hours of quality sleep each night. Create a relaxing bedtime routine, establish a sleep-friendly environment, and practice good sleep hygiene habits.

Prioritize sleep as a non-negotiable part of your daily routine, as it plays a vital role in maintaining optimal health, supporting weight management, and promoting overall well-being.

Embracing a healthy lifestyle also involves adopting.

a positive mindset and cultivating gratitude. Practice self-compassion and focus on self-care rather than self-criticism. Embrace a growth mindset, recognizing that every day is an opportunity for learning, growth, and improvement. Celebrate progress, no matter how small, and acknowledge the effort you put into your health and well-being. Practice gratitude by regularly expressing appreciation for the blessings and positive aspects of your life.

In conclusion, embracing a healthy lifestyle goes beyond weight loss. It encompasses nourishing your body with wholesome foods, engaging in regular physical activity, managing stress effectively, prioritizing self-care, fostering positive relationships, and cultivating a positive mindset.

By adopting a holistic approach to health and well-being, you can enjoy the benefits of a vibrant and fulfilling life well beyond achieving your weight loss goals after

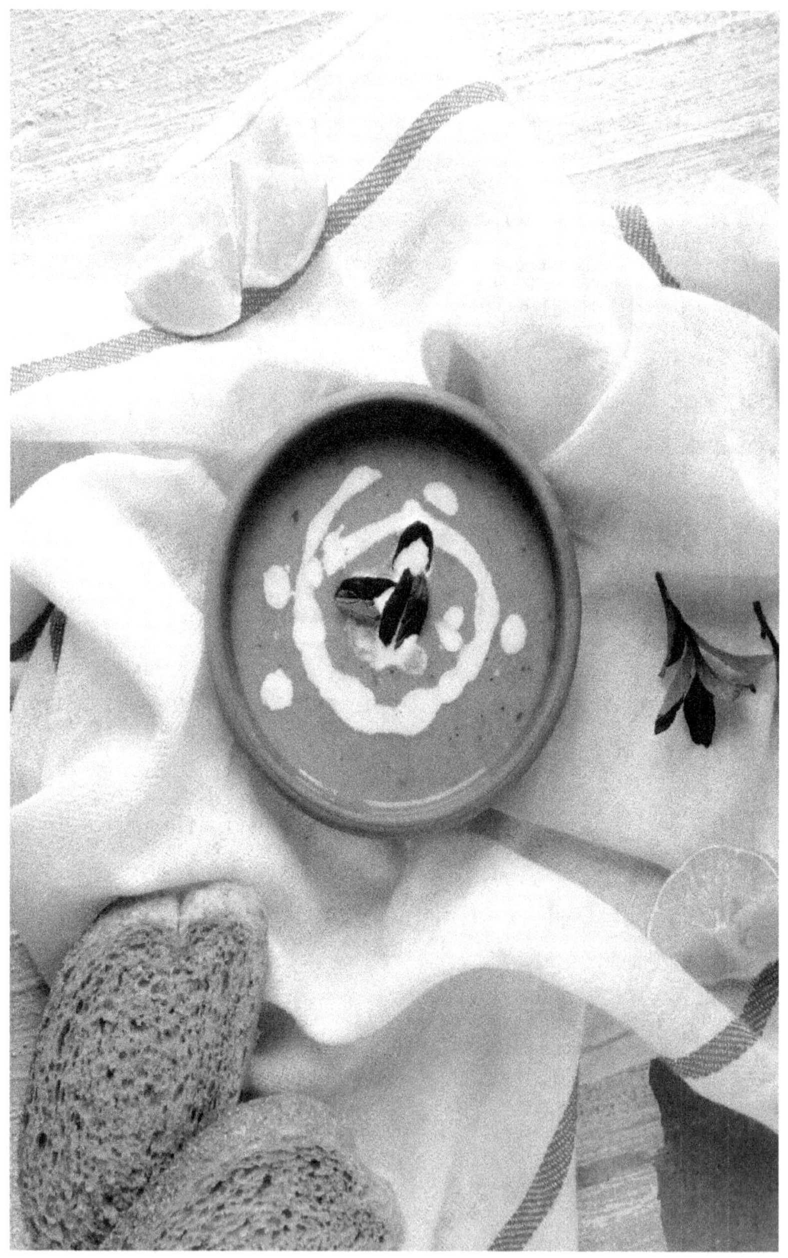

Appendix: Additional Resources

Here are some additional resources that can provide further guidance and support in your journey to losing weight after 50 and maintaining a healthy lifestyle:

Books:

"The Obesity Code" by Dr. Jason Fung

"The Plant-Based Solution" by Dr. Joel Kahn

"The Blue Zones Solution" by Dan Buettner

Online Communities:

MyFitnessPal: A popular online community and app for tracking nutrition and exercise.

SparkPeople: An online community that offers resources, support, and tracking tools for weight loss and healthy living.

Fitness Apps:

MyFitnessPal: Allows you to track your food intake, exercise, and set personalized goals.

Nike Training Club: Provides workout routines and training plans for various fitness levels.

Fitbit: Offers activity tracking, personalized workouts, and sleep monitoring.

Nutrition Websites:

ChooseMyPlate.gov: Provides information on healthy eating, portion sizes, and meal planning.

Academy of Nutrition and Dietetics: Offers resources, articles, and expert advice on nutrition and healthy eating.

Exercise Videos:

Fitness Blender: Provides a wide variety of free workout videos for different fitness levels and goals.

Yoga with Adriene: Offers a collection of yoga videos for all levels, including beginner-friendly routines.

POPSUGAR Fitness: Features a range of workout videos, including cardio, strength training, and dance workouts.

Weight Loss Support Groups:

Weight Watchers: Offers group meetings, online support, and a points-based system for managing food intake.

TOPS (Take Off Pounds Sensibly): Provides local chapter meetings and support for weight loss.

Remember, it's essential to consult with your healthcare provider or a registered dietitian before making any significant changes to your diet or exercise routine. They can offer personalized advice based on your specific needs and medical history.

Note: The resources provided here are for informational purposes only and should not replace professional medical advice. Always consult with a healthcare professional before starting any weight loss or exercise program.

Ten recipes that align with the principles of losing weight after 50 and maintaining a healthy lifestyle:

• Quinoa and Vegetable Salad: A refreshing salad made with protein-rich quinoa, mixed vegetables, herbs, and a light dressing. This recipe provides a balance of nutrients and can be enjoyed as a light lunch or dinner option.

• Baked Salmon with Roasted Vegetables: A delicious and nutritious meal featuring omega-3-rich salmon fillets baked to perfection, accompanied by a colorful assortment of roasted vegetables. This dish is packed with essential nutrients and healthy fats.

• Greek Yogurt Parfait: A satisfying and protein-packed breakfast option consisting of Greek yogurt, fresh berries, nuts, and a drizzle of honey. This recipe provides a balanced combination of macronutrients and antioxidants.

• Veggie Stir-Fry with Tofu: A flavorful stir-fry made with an array of colorful vegetables, tofu, and a savory sauce.

- This recipe is low in calories and high in fiber, making it an ideal choice for weight loss and maintaining a healthy lifestyle.

- Zucchini Noodles with Pesto: A light and low-carb alternative to traditional pasta, zucchini noodles (or "zoodles") are paired with a homemade pesto sauce made from fresh basil, garlic, pine nuts, and olive oil. This recipe is a nutritious and delicious option for a satisfying meal.

- Grilled Chicken Salad with Avocado: A hearty salad featuring grilled chicken breast, mixed greens, cherry tomatoes, cucumbers, and creamy avocado slices. This recipe provides lean protein and healthy fats while being packed with vitamins and minerals.

- Lentil Soup: A comforting and nourishing soup made with lentils, vegetables, and flavorful herbs and spices. This recipe is high in fiber and plant-based protein, making it a filling and nutritious option for a weight-loss-friendly meal.

- Baked Egg Cups with Vegetables: A simple and customizable recipe where eggs are baked in a muffin tin with a variety of vegetables such as spinach, bell peppers, and mushrooms. This recipe is high in protein and low in calories, perfect for a healthy breakfast or snack.

• Turkey Lettuce Wraps: A lighter alternative to traditional wraps, these lettuce wraps feature ground turkey cooked with aromatic spices, topped with crunchy vegetables, and served in lettuce leaves. This recipe is low in carbohydrates and provides lean protein.

• Berry Smoothie Bowl: A colorful and nutrient-packed breakfast option consisting of a blended mixture of frozen berries, a splash of almond milk, and topped with granola, sliced fruits, and seeds. This recipe is rich in antioxidants, vitamins, and fiber.

These recipes highlight a variety of options that are flavorful, satisfying, and in line with the principles of losing weight after 50 and maintaining a healthy lifestyle.

Remember to adjust portion sizes and ingredients based on your individual needs and dietary preferences. Enjoy!

7-day menu plan consisting of breakfast, lunch, and dinner for each day:

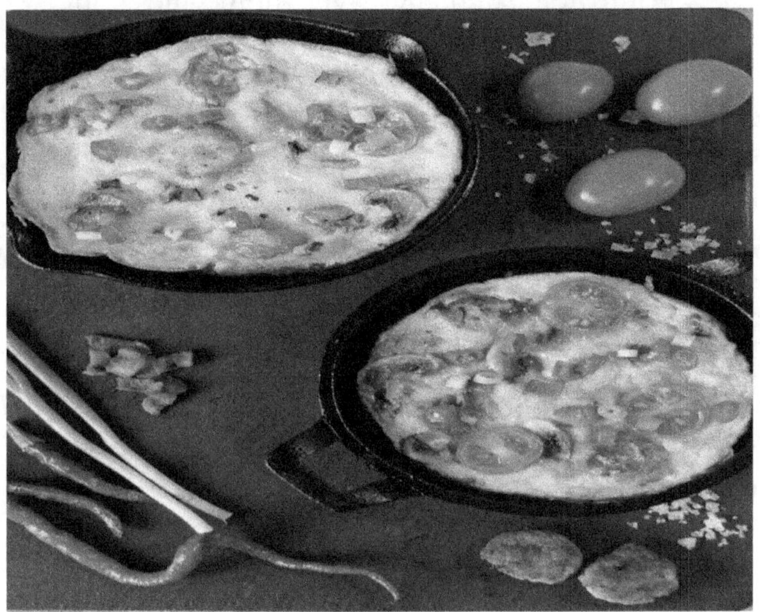

DAY 1

Breakfast: Veggie omelet with Whole Wheat Toast Lunch: Quinoa and Vegetable Salad Dinner: Baked Salmon with Roasted Vegetables

Breakfast: Veggie Omelette with Whole Wheat Toast

Whisk together 3 eggs with a pinch of salt and black pepper.

Heat a non-stick pan over medium heat and coat with cooking spray.

Add diced bell peppers, onions, and spinach to the pan and sauté until tender.

Pour the beaten eggs over the veggies and cook until the edges are set.

Carefully flip the Omelette and cook for another minute or until fully cooked.

Serve the Omelette with a slice of whole wheat toast.

Lunch: Quinoa and Vegetable Salad

Cook 1/2 cup of quinoa according to package instructions and let it cool.

In a large bowl, combine the cooked quinoa with chopped cucumbers, cherry tomatoes, bell peppers, red onions, and fresh herbs like parsley and mint.

Drizzle with a light vinaigrette made with olive oil, lemon juice, salt, and pepper.

Toss everything together until well combined.

Optional: Add grilled chicken or tofu for added protein.

Dinner: Baked Salmon with Roasted Vegetables

Preheat the oven to 400°F (200°C).

Season salmon fillets with salt, pepper, and a squeeze of lemon juice.

Place the salmon on a baking sheet lined with parchment paper and bake for about 12-15 minutes or until cooked through and flaky.

While the salmon is baking, prepare the roasted vegetables.

Toss asparagus spears and cherry tomatoes with olive oil, garlic, salt, and pepper.

Arrange the vegetables on another baking sheet and roast for about 10-12 minutes or until tender.

Serve the baked salmon with the roasted vegetables and a side of your choice, such as quinoa or brown rice.

Feel free to customize the portions and adjust the ingredients according to your preferences. Enjoy your nutritious and delicious meals!

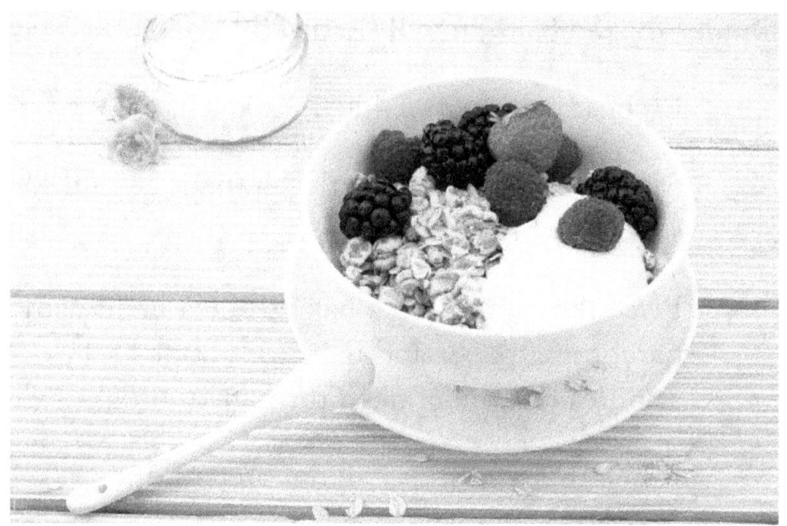

DAY 2

Breakfast: Greek Yogurt Parfait with Fresh Berries and Granola Lunch: Turkey Lettuce Wraps Dinner: Chicken Stir-Fry with Brown Rice

Breakfast: Greek Yogurt Parfait with Fresh Berries and Granola

In a glass or bowl, layer Greek yogurt, fresh berries (such as strawberries, blueberries, and raspberries), and a sprinkle of granola.

Repeat the layers until you reach your desired amount.

Optional: Drizzle a small amount of honey or maple syrup for added sweetness.

Lunch: Turkey Lettuce Wraps

Cook ground turkey in a skillet until browned and cooked through.

Add minced garlic, diced onions, and chopped bell peppers to the skillet and sauté until vegetables are tender.

Season with your preferred spices, such as cumin, paprika, and chili powder.

Serve the turkey mixture in lettuce leaves, such as butter lettuce or romaine hearts.

Optional: Top with diced tomatoes, avocado slices, and a squeeze of lime juice.

Dinner: Chicken Stir-Fry with Brown Rice

Heat a tablespoon of oil in a large pan or wok over medium-high heat.

Add diced chicken breast and cook until browned and cooked through.

Remove the chicken from the pan and set aside.

In the same pan, add sliced bell peppers, broccoli florets, sliced carrots, and any other desired vegetables.

Stir-fry the vegetables until crisp-tender.

Return the cooked chicken to the pan and add a stir-fry sauce of your choice (e.g., soy sauce, ginger, garlic, and a splash of honey).

Cook for a few more minutes until the flavors are well combined.

Serve the chicken stir-fry over a bed of cooked brown rice.

Feel free to adjust the portions and ingredients to suit your preferences. Enjoy your nutritious and flavorful meals!

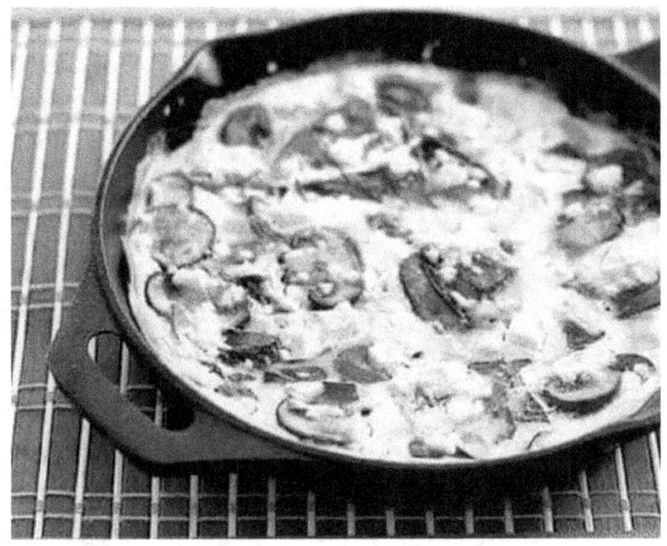

DAY 3

Breakfast: Spinach and Mushroom Frittata Lunch: Lentil Soup with Whole Grain Bread Dinner: Grilled Chicken Breast with Steamed Broccoli and Sweet Potato Mas

Breakfast: Spinach and Mushroom Frittata

Preheat the oven to 375°F (190°C).

In an oven-safe skillet, sauté sliced mushrooms and chopped spinach until wilted.

In a separate bowl, whisk together eggs, salt, pepper, and a splash of milk.

Pour the egg mixture over the sautéed.

vegetables

Cook on the stovetop over medium heat for a few minutes until the edges start to set.

Transfer the skillet to the preheated oven and bake for about 15-20 minutes or until the frittata is set and golden brown on top. Slice into wedges and serve.

Lunch: Lentil Soup with Whole Grain Bread

In a large pot, heat some olive oil and sauté chopped onions, minced garlic, and diced carrots until tender.

Add rinsed lentils, vegetable broth, diced tomatoes, and your choice of herbs and spices (such as cumin, paprika, and thyme).

Bring the soup to a boil, then reduce the heat and simmer for about 30-40 minutes until the lentils are tender.

Season with salt and pepper to taste.

Serve the lentil soup with a side of whole grain bread for dipping.

Dinner: Grilled Chicken Breast with Steamed Broccoli and Sweet Potato Mash

Preheat the grill to medium-high heat.

Season chicken breast with salt, pepper, and your preferred seasonings (such as garlic powder, paprika, and dried herbs).

Grill the chicken for about 6-8 minutes per side or until cooked through.

Meanwhile, steam broccoli florets until tender-crisp.

In a separate pot, boil peeled and cubed sweet potatoes until soft.

Drain the sweet potatoes and mash them with a little butter or olive oil, a splash of milk, and a pinch of salt and pepper.

Serve the grilled chicken breast with steamed broccoli and a scoop of sweet potato mash.

Feel free to adjust the portions and ingredients based on your preferences. Enjoy your nutritious and satisfying meals!

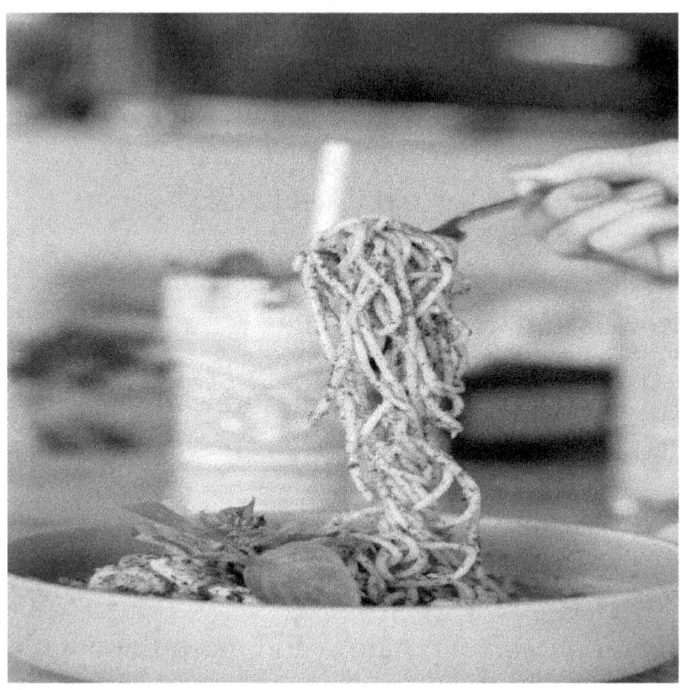

DAY 4

Breakfast: Overnight Chia Pudding with Mixed Berries Lunch: Zucchini Noodles with Pesto and Grilled Shrimp Dinner: Baked Cod with Lemon Butter Sauce, Quinoa Pilaf, and Roasted Brussels Sprouts

Breakfast: Overnight Chia Pudding with Mixed Berries

In a jar or bowl, combine chia seeds, your choice of milk (such as almond milk or coconut milk), a sweetener like maple syrup or honey, and a splash of vanilla extract.

Stir well to ensure the chia seeds are evenly distributed.

Cover and refrigerate overnight or for at least 4 hours until the mixture thickens, and the chia seeds absorb the liquid.

In the morning, give the chia pudding a good stir and top with a variety of mixed berries, such as strawberries, blueberries, and raspberries.

Optional: Sprinkle with a handful of chopped nuts or a drizzle of nut butter for added crunch and flavor.

Lunch: Zucchini Noodles with Pesto and Grilled Shrimp

Use a spiralizer or julienne peeler to create zucchini noodles (zoodles) from fresh zucchini.

In a pan, heat some olive oil and sauté the zucchini noodles for a few minutes until just tender.

Meanwhile, prepare the pesto sauce by blending fresh basil leaves, pine nuts, garlic, grated Parmesan cheese, and olive oil until smooth. Adjust the consistency and seasoning to your liking.

Grill shrimp until cooked through and lightly charred.

Toss the zucchini noodles with the pesto sauce and top with the grilled shrimp.

Optional: Sprinkle with extra Parmesan cheese or a squeeze of lemon juice.

Dinner: Baked Cod with Lemon Butter Sauce, Quinoa Pilaf, and Roasted Brussels Sprouts

Preheat the oven to 375°F (190°C).

Place cod fillets on a baking sheet lined with parchment paper.

In a small bowl, mix melted butter, lemon Juice, minced garlic, and chopped parsley. Brush the mixture over the cod fillets.

Bake for about 12-15 minutes or until the cod is cooked through and flakes easily with a fork.

While the cod is baking, cook quinoa.

according to package instructions and fluff with a fork.

For the quinoa pilaf, sauté diced onions, bell peppers, and a handful of mixed vegetables in a pan until softened. Stir in the cooked quinoa and season with salt, pepper, and your choice of herbs.

Toss Brussels sprouts with olive oil, salt, and pepper, and roast in the oven until golden and tender.

Serve the baked cod with a drizzle of lemon butter sauce, alongside the quinoa pilaf and roasted Brussels sprouts.

Feel free to adjust the portions and ingredients according to your preferences. Enjoy your delicious and wholesome meals.

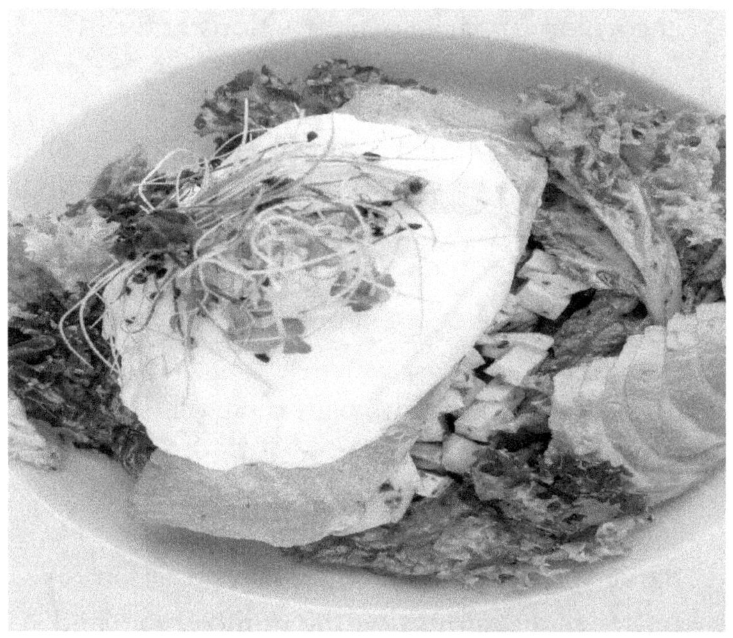

DAY 5

Breakfast: Avocado Toast with Poached Eggs
Lunch: Chickpea Salad with Mixed Greens Dinner:
Vegetable Curry with Brown Rice

Breakfast: Avocado Toast with Poached Eggs

Toast whole grain bread slices until golden and crispy.

Mash ripe avocado with a squeeze of lemon juice, salt, and pepper.

Spread the mashed avocado on the toasted bread slices.

Top each slice with a perfectly poached egg.

Optional: Sprinkle with red pepper flakes or chopped fresh herbs like cilantro or parsley.

Lunch: Chickpea Salad with Mixed Greens

In a large bowl, combine mixed salad greens, drained and rinsed canned chickpeas, diced cucumbers, cherry tomatoes, sliced red onions, and chopped fresh herbs like parsley or mint.

Toss the salad with a simple dressing made of olive oil, lemon juice, salt, and pepper.

Optional: Add crumbled feta cheese or sliced avocado for extra flavor and creaminess.

Dinner: Vegetable Curry with Brown Rice

In a large pot, heat some oil and sauté diced onions, minced garlic, and grated ginger until fragrant.

Add your choice of mixed vegetables, such as bell peppers, carrots, cauliflower, and green beans. Cook until slightly tender.

Stir in curry powder, turmeric, cumin, and coriander, and cook for another minute to release the flavors.

Pour in coconut milk and vegetable broth and let the curry simmer for about 15-20 minutes until the vegetables are cooked through.

Season with salt, pepper, and a squeeze of lime juice to taste.

Serve the vegetable curry over cooked brown rice.

Feel free to adjust the portions and ingredients to suit your preferences. Enjoy your flavorful and nourishing meals!

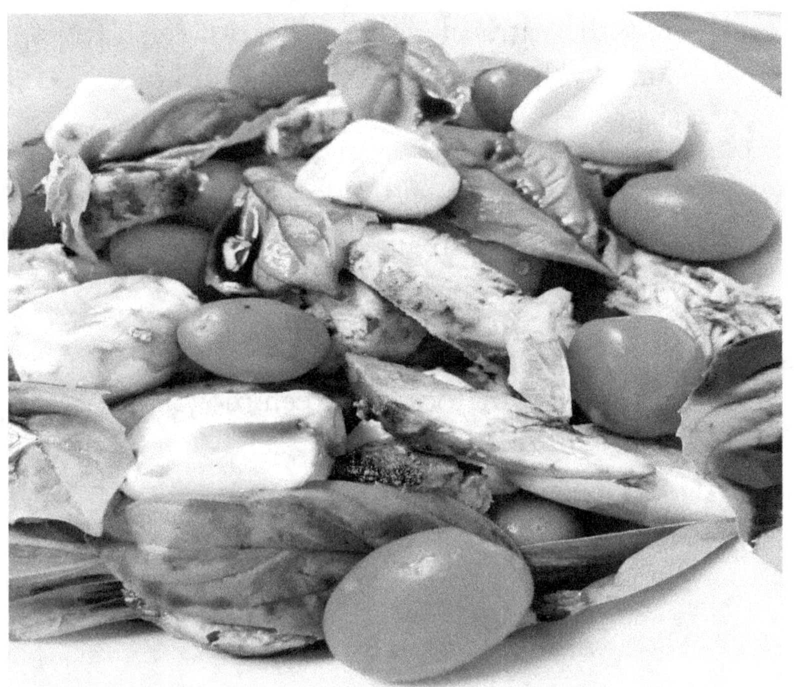

DAY 6

Breakfast: Oatmeal with Fresh Fruit and Almonds
Lunch: Caprese Salad with Grilled Chicken Dinner:
Beef Stir-Fry with Broccoli and Cauliflower Rice

Breakfast: Oatmeal with Fresh Fruit and Almonds

Cook rolled oats with your choice of milk
(such as almond milk or oat milk)
according to package instructions.

Once cooked, stir in a drizzle of honey or
maple syrup for sweetness.

Top the oatmeal with a variety of fresh fruits, such as sliced bananas, berries, and diced apples.

Sprinkle with a handful of chopped almonds for added crunch and protein.

Lunch: Caprese Salad with Grilled Chicken

Slice ripe tomatoes and fresh mozzarella cheese into rounds.

Arrange the tomato and mozzarella slices on a plate, alternating them.

Top with fresh basil leaves.

Drizzle with balsamic glaze or reduction, and a drizzle of extra virgin

olive oil.

Grill chicken breast until cooked through and slice into strips.

Place the grilled chicken strips on top of the caprese salad.

Season with salt, pepper, and a sprinkle of dried oregano.

Dinner: Beef Stir-Fry with Broccoli and Cauliflower Rice

Slice beef steak into thin strips.

In a hot pan or wok, stir-fry the beef strips with a little oil until browned and cooked to your liking.

Remove the beef from the pan and set aside.

In the same pan, stir-fry broccoli florets and cauliflower rice until tender-crisp.

Return the cooked beef to the pan and add a stir-fry sauce made of soy sauce, minced garlic, grated ginger, and a touch of honey.

Cook for a few more minutes until the flavors meld together.

Optional: Garnish with sliced green onions or sesame seeds for added flavor and presentation.

Feel free to adjust the portions and ingredients based on your preferences. Enjoy your nutritious and delicious meals!

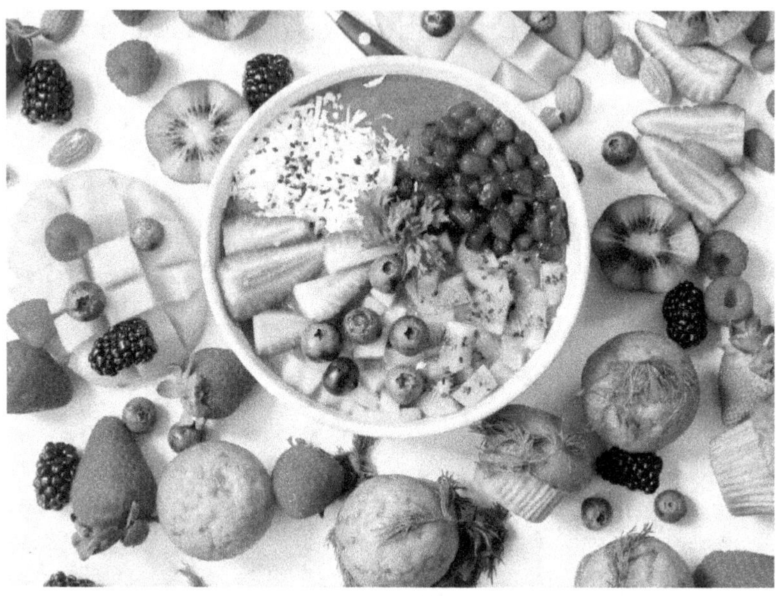

DAY 7

Breakfast: Whole Grain Pancakes with Maple Syrup and Fresh Berries Lunch: Quinoa Stuffed Bell Peppers Dinner: Baked Chicken Thighs with Roasted Asparagus and Garlic Herb Mashed Potatoes

Breakfast: Smoothie Bowl with Toppings

> In a blender, blend frozen mixed berries, a ripe banana, Greek yogurt, and a splash of almond milk until smooth and creamy.

> Pour the smoothie into a bowl.

Top the smoothie bowl with a variety of toppings, such as sliced fresh fruits (e.g., kiwi, mango, and berries), granola, chia seeds, and a drizzle of nut butter.

Lunch: Quinoa and Black Bean Salad

Cook quinoa according to package instructions and let it cool.

In a large bowl, combine cooked quinoa, rinsed and drained black beans, diced bell peppers, diced red onions, chopped cilantro, and corn kernels.

Drizzle with a zesty dressing made of lime juice, olive oil, minced garlic, cumin, and a pinch of salt and pepper.

Toss everything together until well combined.

Optional: Add diced avocado or crumbled feta cheese for added creaminess.

Dinner: Grilled Vegetable Skewers with Herbed Couscous

Preheat the grill to medium heat.

Cut a variety of vegetables into bite-sized pieces, such as bell peppers, zucchini, eggplant, cherry tomatoes, and red onions.

Thread the vegetables onto skewers.

Brush the skewers with olive oil and season with salt, pepper, and your preferred herbs, such as oregano or thyme.

Grill the vegetable skewers, turning occasionally, until they are tender and slightly charred.

While the skewers are grilling, prepare herbed couscous by cooking couscous according to package instructions and stirring in chopped fresh herbs like parsley and mint.

Serve the grilled vegetable skewers with a side of herbed couscous.

Note: Feel free to adjust portion sizes and ingredients according to your dietary needs and preferences. It is always good to incorporate a variety of fruits, vegetables, lean proteins, and whole grains into your meals for a well-balanced and nutritious diet.

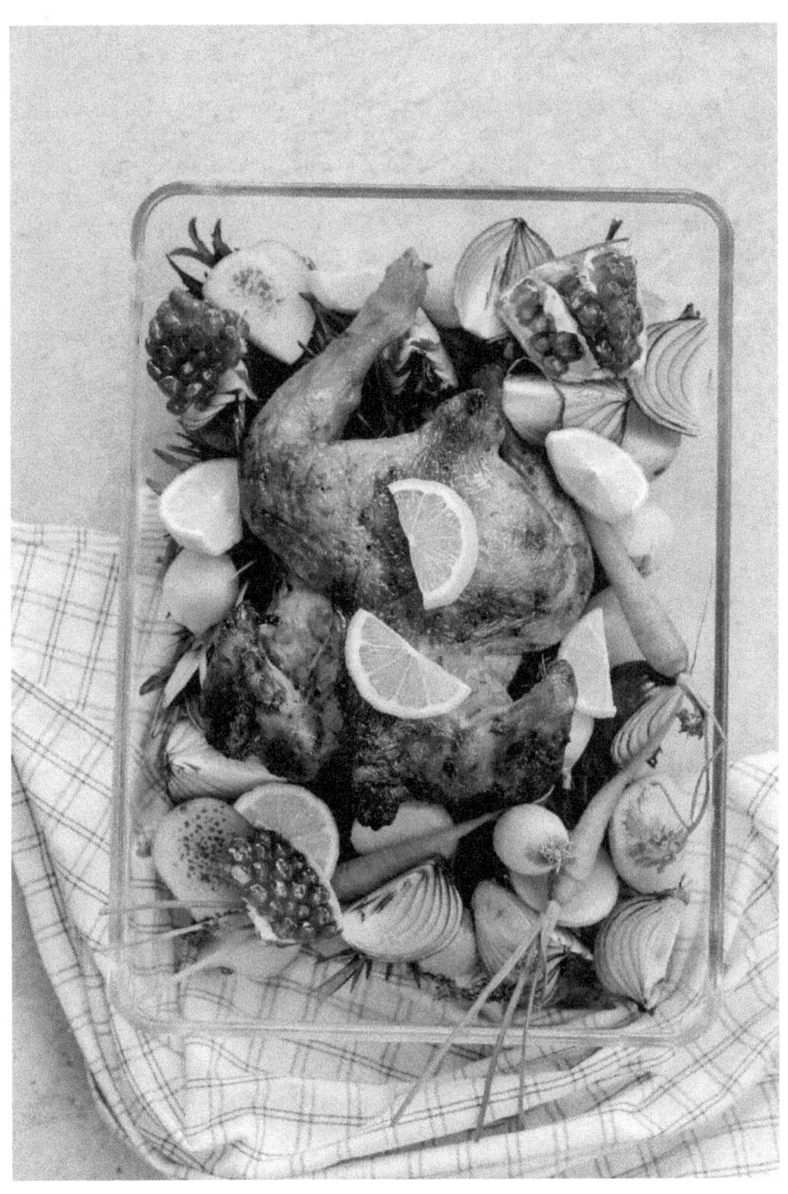

ABOUT THE AUTHOR

Olive Antoine is a wife and mother who experienced a noticeable change in her weight after turning fifty years old. She developed difficulty with menopause and a slow thyroid. After many failed attempts at weight loss, she found the right mix of exercise, diet, and lifestyle changes that enabled her to experience and maintain significant weight loss. This book reflects her experience, and she hopes it will help others to find their true self again.